RHEUMATISM, POLYARTHRITIS, AND OTHER JOINT DISEASE

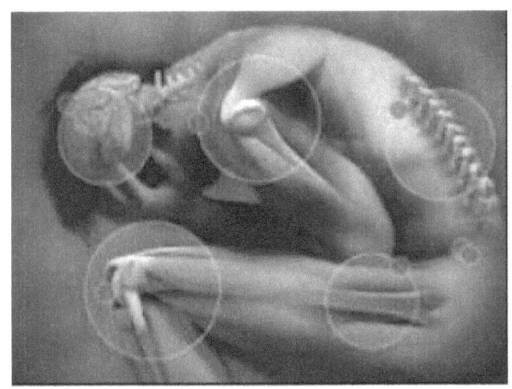

ARTHRITIS IS NOT INCURABLE

By Kerri Ryan

www.Nutritional-Therapy.us

Contents

RHEUMATISM, POLYARTHRITIS, AND OTHER JOINT DISEASE 1

RA, Rheumatism, and Joint Pain All Stem From the Same Problem 2

ARTHRITIS OVERVIEW 5

TOO MANY NAMES FOR THE SAME THING 9

HERBAL MEDICINES; MAYBE, MAYBE NOT 11

IMPORTANT TO REMEMBER 13

CORTICOSTEROIDS, ACTH, and ASPIRIN 15

CORTICOSTEROID TREATMENTS 17

ASPIRIN 20

A DISEASE OF ADRENAL EXHAUSTION 22

VITAMIN C AND PANTOTHENIC ACID (VITAMIN B5) . 24

VITAMIN C 27

HOW MUCH VITAMIN C IS ENOUGH? 27

PROTEIN AND FATTY ACIDS 30

WHY SO LITTLE REFERRANCE TO VITAMINS AND MINERALS? 31

OSTEOARTHRITIS AND ITS RELATION TO MAGNESIUM, CALCIUM, AND VITAMIN E 32

PHOSPHEROUS 35

SUMMARY 36

Nutritional Therapy's Medical Disclaimer; 39

RA, Rheumatism, and Joint Pain All Stem From the Same Problem

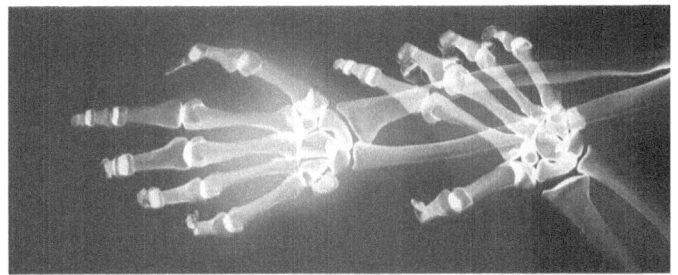

There have been lots of controversy over arthritis treatments, and there is little wonder why. Wherever you go; MAYO Clinic, National Institutes of Health, NY Times Health section (don't laugh, many people rely on this), even the National Arthritis Foundation will all tell you that there is no cure for arthritis, but only ways to manage it; primarily with drugs. The majority of mainstream resources that we go through don't even mention vitamins and minerals, with the exception of the Arthritis Foundation, and even this was inconclusive.

The appalling lack of research on vitamins and minerals doesn't seem to be any accident. Seeing how pharmaceutical companies are funding most of the medical research and medical colleges in this country, it is easy to see why they would not want to support the competition.

Back in the 40's, and 50's, there was a great deal of arthritis research done with nutrition, and it produced some amazingly positive results. However, with the immediate relief and availability drugs had to offer, the public mindset drifted towards drug use and pain relievers instead. Not so long ago, doctors were a walking billboard for the pharmaceutical companies, handing out samples, prescribing exclusive prescriptions, and even wearing 'donated' equipment with 'big pharm' advertisements plastered all over them. This influence over healing became so intrusive that new laws were passed in the beginning of 2012 that severely limits the role pharmaceutical reps have when they visit practicing doctors.[1]

Diet and nutrition were the standard forms of medical treatment for centuries until the discovery of penicillin by Alexander Fleming in 1928.[2] During the US Civil War, more soldiers died of infection than injury, so penicillin became the wonder drug that set the pace for the next several generations, even until today. When Jonas Salk's vaccine for polio was determined a success on April 12, 1955[3], as it rightly deserves, the notion of 'drugs' was firmly established as the primary way to treat illness and disease from that point forward. Please don't misunderstand- vaccines and pharmacological drugs for infectious and contagious diseases are a necessity for modern medicine and should not be done away with. The immediate treatment these drugs provide is a staple in the medical industry, around the world. However, when it comes to long term, metabolic diseases that develop over time, these need to be addressed from the inside out by restoring the body's natural ability to heal itself.

With health care costs spiraling out of control, and drug related treatments leaving people with more problems than they started out with, more and more people are searching for more natural ways to regain their health. They are returning to vitamins and minerals simply because they need answers that they are not getting from main stream medicine. People are becoming increasingly challenged to pay for these treatments, and not getting enough good results. Traditional pharmacological treatments are now costing people too much, in more ways than one. The main reason for this shift is simply because nutrition works.

With such bleak stats surrounding arthritis and all its forms, it can leave anyone feeling defeated, adding to the stress of the disease. However, this eBook will explain how there are several ways to reverse inflammation and swelling; ways to stop this progressive disease, and for some, ways to eliminate it altogether. There are even records of those with scar tissue and fused bone that have had miraculous results from diet and exercise alone.[4] It doesn't happen overnight, and there is no magic bullet, but by focusing on a few specific nutritional elements, anyone can experience at least improvement, if not remission altogether.

ARTHRITIS OVERVIEW

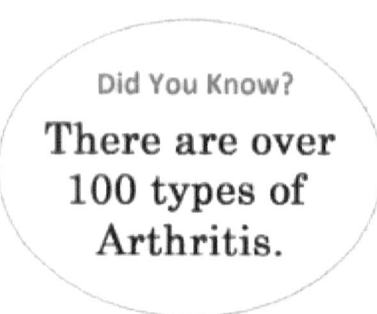

Did You Know?
There are over 100 types of Arthritis.

According to the American Arthritis Foundation, there are over 100 different types of arthritis that are named; affecting approximately 46 million people in the United States alone.[5] The financial impact of arthritis on society is by some estimates $128 billion annually[6]. Those suffering from this increasing problem have grown from 35 million in 1985, to 43 million in 2006, affecting 1 in 5 adults, and almost 300,000 children.[7] Arthritis is one of the most rampant chronic health issues in the United States, and the primary cause of disability among people over the age of 15.[8]

Despite the fact that research has proven how diet and exercise will reduce and even eliminate the symptoms of arthritis, mainstream medicine is slow to accept these facts. The focus of this eBook will be to explain arthritis, and the ways the body reacts to it; and then offer solutions on how to reverse the process. Since there are so many varieties, effecting all areas of the body, I want to put arthritis in perspective first.

The treatment of inflammation can include everything from Acetaminophen, to joint replacement, but some of the most common treatments and therapies will include the following;

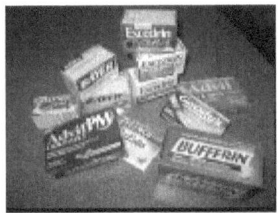

*Over the counter anti-inflammatory drugs; however, these can cause cardiovascular problems, liver and kidney trouble, bleeding ulcers, and a ringing in your ears; especially in older people. There is not really much difference between these and a low-grade narcotic.

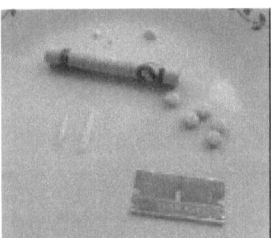

*Prescription drugs including narcotics; narcotics can easily become addictive which unfortunately some people are willing to risk if their pain is severe enough. Other side effects can include drowsiness, constipation, and digestive issues.

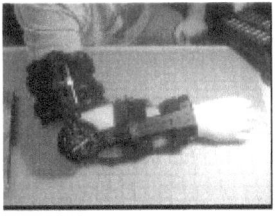

*Braces and other support devices can be helpful at the onset of arthritis, but they are certainly no way to live. These are very limiting, and do nothing to improve the overall condition. If someone's pain is so severe that support systems are needed, then by all means use them, but it is our hope that this eBook will show you how to gradually reduce the pain of arthritis to the point that painless, fluid movement becomes your standard once again.

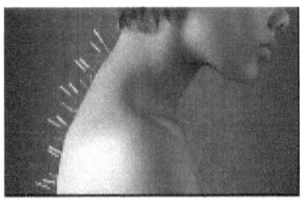

*Acupuncture- This ancient form of medicine does offer relief, but at a price. As the needle punctures the skin, it triggers a chain reaction in the body. As with a bee sting, the body will throw up a wall of water to contain whatever chemical toxin broke through the skin, and then go about trying to remove it from the body. This process will cause the adrenal glands to release chemicals that will help to reduce swelling and inflammation, including those associated with arthritis. However, in the end it leaves the adrenal glands more exhausted than they were at the start. Like other anti-inflammatory drugs, acupuncture is forcing the body to do what it should be doing if it were strong and healthy. Acupuncture is good for a short-term relief but will actually add more stress to the body in the long run.

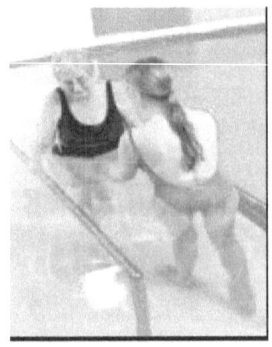

*Physical therapy; this is probably the best form of

treatment, but only if the body has enough nutrients to rebuild itself after the stresses of exercise have been placed on it. Anyone with severe, or even mild joint pain, should gradually work up to a physical therapy regimen, after they give their body the nutrition it needs. Making sure that the patient is eating a targeted diet designed to reduce swelling and inflammation, and build up the body's ability to combat stress no matter where it flares up, should be the goal of those who want arthritis relief. When exercise is practiced with this kind of diet; exercise will be one of the best treatments for arthritis that there is.

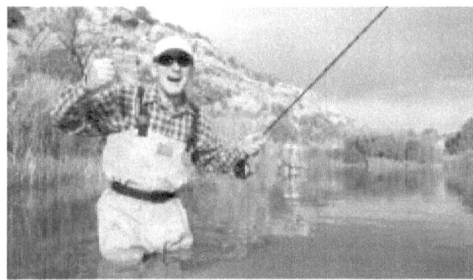

*Hobbies; Relieving mental stress with a hobby, or some form of exercise is as equally important as relieving physical stress. As any good doctor will tell you, exercise is always good. However, what we are saying is that any exercise is good, but having a parallel amount of nutrition to go along with it is exponentially better. Stress has a tremendous impact on the body and causes it to release countless chemicals that can either make or break a person. Limiting the impact of stress- mental & physical- is what this book is all about. It will take a look at what goes on at the cellular level, and talk about what the body needs to reduce swelling and inflammation, and how to get this process started as soon as possible.

TOO MANY NAMES FOR THE SAME THING

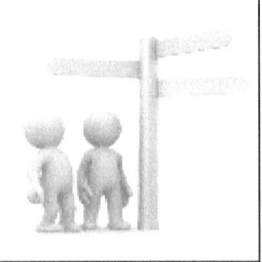

With so many types of 'arthritis' being labeled to every ache and pain that we may experience, it can be overwhelming for some to get a straight answer. What most people need is to get answers on how to relieve their specific issue, without being drawn into a world of diseases, drugs, expense, and everyone talking a new and completely different language. All most people know is that they hurt, and they want the pain to stop. Unlike the mainstream medical industry, Nutritional-Therapy Medicine will not try to treat the symptom, but rather go right after the cause. Instead of chasing 3 or 4 different types of arthritis that add up to a person feeling terrible, we are going to look at what causes inflammation in general- no matter where it is- and how to build up your body so that it can self-correct itself enough to produce real, lasting results.

By looking at the body as a whole; and how the body responds to stress, Alternative Medicine will focus on what the body needs to perform naturally, without the aid of synthetic drugs. Results are clear; relief can be found; it is being found; and it can be found by you.

None of the recommendations here will contradict any drugs or meds that a person may already be taking, however, since everyone is unique, we always suggest that our readers take this advice along with the advice of their personal doctor. Research has shown that there is no "1" perfect answer to reduce the inflammation of joints, but it will take a few things that work together to reduce swelling and restore painless, fluid movement.

Building up the adrenal glands is often, one of the first things considered with any disease, and we will dedicate an entire chapter as to how and why this works. For arthritic patients, this alone will allow them to produce their own cortisone, so they can eventually stop taking synthetic supplements.

HERBAL MEDICINES; MAYBE, MAYBE NOT

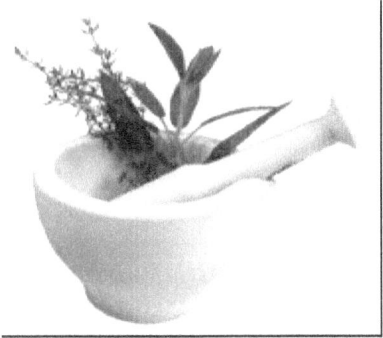

There seems to be a general prejudice against alternative medicine that believes it is comprised of herbalists, and those who rely on ancient remedies, and backyard tinctures to cure every disease known to man. While herbs can also play an important role in healing, we considered them to be good food, but should not be relied on too heavily. There are too many 'snake oil salesmen' out there who will tout the benefits of the dandelion root, Ginkgo, or St. John's Wart to solve any ailment that comes along. All of these claims likely have some merit to them, or they would not have remained in their prominent place around the world like they have. However, Nutritional-Therapy would like to know exactly what is it about the dandelion root, Ginkgo and St. John's Wart- or any herb- that produces a positive response.

For this reason, we will not be considering herbal remedies, but rather looking at the vitamins and minerals within herbs and learning more about what role each one plays. It is not our belief that by randomly adding various naturally occurring plants to the diet is an acceptable form of treatment. For those suffering from severely debilitating diseases, taking herbal remedies on the chance that it will reduce their pain, and reverse their condition is not enough to stand on. There is more than one factor behind the cause of all diseases, and therefore their solutions cannot be found in one remedy alone.

By researching the effects of vitamins and minerals on a cellular level, and discovering what elements impact what part of the body, we will show how these studies have produced some amazing results; most of which if maintained, will last a lifetime. Even diseases that have left people with scar tissue and fused bones have been known to reverse themselves in some extreme cases.[9] There is always hope of improvement, and sometimes there is even more.

IMPORTANT TO REMEMBER

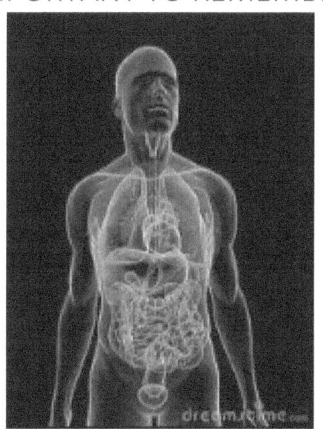

When treating arthritis, or any disease with vitamins and minerals, decades of people have found that other symptoms they were suffering from have also gradually disappeared, too. Like all reputable organizations, Nutritional Therapy respects the whole person, and the fact that their unique situation should be viewed on an individual basis. The body and its workings are extremely complex and should be treated as unique parts working together along with the mental and emotional aspects of every human being.

Since many illnesses stem from stress, reducing it is paramount to healing. When the body is under stress it will release excessive amounts of Cortisol, that will actively damage the tissues of the body. Chronic stress can bring on heart disease, diabetes, and even cancer.[10] This is particularly true when dealing with a victim of arthritis. The stress of chronic pain has more effects on the body than just being uncomfortable. It is important to remember that;

1. "Each person is an individual and should be viewed as a person with a type of arthritis, rather than as a type of arthritis; with a person.

2. There is no 'one' treatment for everyone who has an arthritis, as each individual may respond differently to various treatments.

3. No single type of arthritis is better or worse than another.

4. Information and input from a person with arthritis is as valuable in diagnosis and management as information from laboratory tests and X-rays.

5. In arthritis management, the emphasis is on improving function of joints and relieving pain.

6. Your involvement, plus that of your doctor are fully needed to help you. People with arthritis and health professionals are partners in care.

7. Something can always be done to improve the situation for a person with arthritis."[11]

While great strides have been made in the field of arthritis over the years, none is more positive than mainstream medicine's acceptance of supplemental help from other sources. As the American Arthritis Foundation states;

> "One of the most exciting changes in recent years has been the growing understanding that the patient has an important role to play in the management of his or her arthritis. This change in emphasis is sometimes referred to as a 'bio-psycho-social'[12] model of disease management, to distinguish it from the traditional biomedical model, in which the outcomes of diseases are thought to be determined almost exclusively by the actions of health professionals.
>
> The wonderful advances in [medical treatments] are an important component of a biopsychosocial model of disease management, but this model also incorporates the key contribution of patients, families and support networks to the outcome."[13] [Emphasis added]

By working together with other forms of effective treatment, doctors are beginning to realize that drugs alone are not the answer. They only treat the symptom; not the cause.

CORTICOSTEROIDS, ACTH, and ASPIRIN

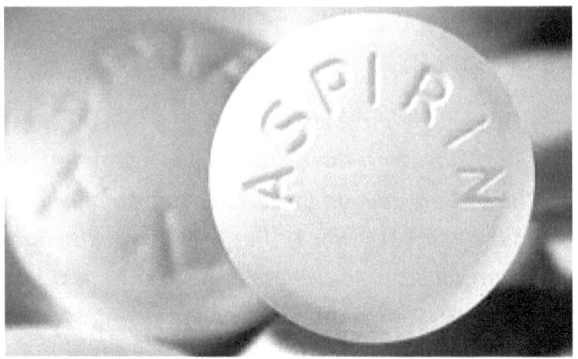

Some of the most popular forms of arthritis treatment include

*Cortisone therapy

*ACTH (Adrenocorticotropic hormone) therapy, and

*Aspirin

Vitamins and minerals will not interfere with any of these treatment plans, but these synthetic treatments will hinder the effects of vitamins and minerals. The goal here would be to get the body producing its own anti-inflammatory chemicals as it was designed to do. Once the body is replenished naturally, the patient and their doctor can gradually wean themselves off synthetic drugs as their condition improves. We cannot make blanket statements here, as each patient is unique; but we will explain how the body responds to all the various substances, and hopefully that will help you make the best decision for you.

It is a prevailing thought within mainstream medicine that by suppressing the body's natural defense mechanisms, and applying man-made drugs, that this will eventually lead to healing. In Truth, these procedures will only mask the real problem and treat the symptoms, making us feel better until a more permanent solution shows up. Aspirin is a classic example. Aspirin suppresses the prostaglandins in order to block pain[14], but it does nothing to stop it.

Steroids and ACTH will suppress inflammation but do nothing to restore the body's natural anti-inflammatory process. In fact; long term use of steroids will suppress the body enough to cause permanent damage.[15]

While these procedures provide tremendous immediate relief for the patient, when produced synthetically they lack a certain something that allows them to operate smoothly, long term, and without side effects.

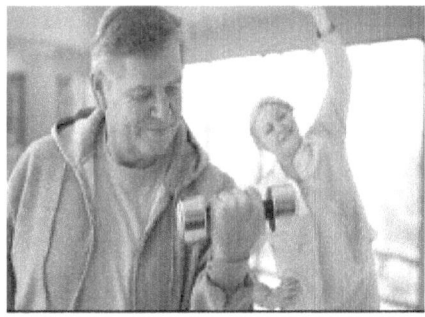

CORTICOSTEROID TREATMENTS

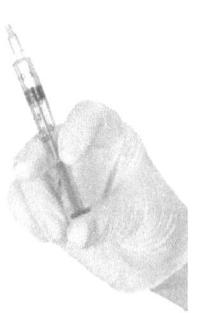

Some of the injection pictures I was considering for this chapter were just too painful to look at- yet that is the reality. Steroid shots are painful and have several side effects.[16] Complications can include;

- Joint infection
- Nerve damage
- Thinning of skin and soft tissue around the injection site
- Temporary flare of pain and inflammation in the joint
- Tendon weakening or rupture
- Thinning of nearby bone (osteoporosis)
- Whitening or lightening of the skin around the injection site
- Death of nearby bone (osteonecrosis)
- Temporary increase in blood sugar

The adrenal glands are situated on top of the kidneys. They produce some of the most important chemicals that the body needs to remain healthy, including cortisone, hydrocortisone and prednisone. These hormones affect many diseases besides arthritis, including allergies and asthma. When produced naturally, there are no side effects associated with them. When produced synthetically and introduced into the body, they can include all those listed side effects including a suppressed immune system; making you even more susceptible to diseases of all kinds.

Corticosteroids are known to cause; first and foremost suppressed adrenal glands function. As said before, this will make us feel better at the onset, but long term use will leave us worse off than we were before we started taking them. They give an immediate but temporary relief from pain, but in the end they place an even greater amount of stress on the overall body in addition to the already weakened adrenals. This path is the same as effectively whipping a dead horse.

ACTH (Adreno-cortico-tropic hormone) is a hormone secreted by the pituitary gland within the brain. It is an important component of the hypothalamic-pituitary-adrenal axis (HPA axis), believed to be the center of the neuro-endocrine system. Hormones that come from these glands control reactions to stress and regulate many body processes, besides those related to arthritis.[17]

ACTH is a very powerful hormone that has been researched for decades, all over the world, and rarely more completely than by the Children's Hospital, Helsinki, and the Aurora Hospital, also in Helsinki, Finland. This report by the National Institutes of Health, Washington, DC shows that;

> "162 children with infantile spasms were treated with ACTH at the Children's Hospital[18], Helsinki, and at the Aurora Hospital, Helsinki... In a large proportion (37%) of the children with treatment caused pronounced side effects, and the mortality was 4.9%. The most common complications were infections: septic infections, pneumonias, and urinary and gastrointestinal infections. Other side effects were arterial hypertension[19], osteoporosis[20], hypokalemic alkalosis[21], and other marked electrolyte disturbances[22]. In children necropsy showed

fresh intracerebral hemorrhages. Four children developed oliguria and hyperkalemia during and after withdrawal of ACTH. One of them had tubular necrosis confirmed by renal biopsy. Infections were significantly more common with large doses (120 units) of ACTH than with small ones (40 units). It is concluded that side effects, even severe ones, are more common during treatment than had been assumed. Careful watch is important before and after treatment. The benefit of very high dosages should also be reconsidered."[23]

While hormone therapy is a welcome short-term relief for constant pain and discomfort, clearly it can cause far more damage than good when taken synthetically over an extended period of time.

ASPIRIN

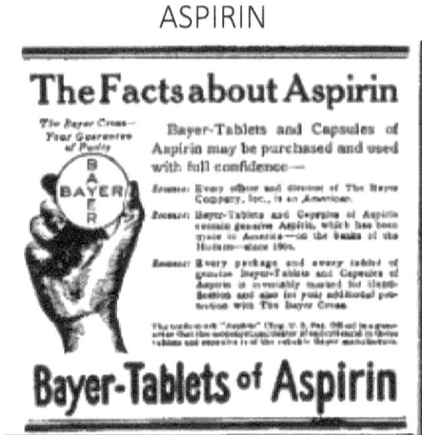

Aspirin is part of the salicylates family of chemicals. They have been known for centuries, first recorded by Hippocrates in the 5th century, B.C. He wrote about a bitter powder extracted from willow bark that could ease aches and pains and reduce fevers. Today's research has shown that part of the willow bark that produces these results is called 'salicin', hence the name 'salicylates'.

When the body experiences pain, it sends chemicals called 'prostaglandins' to the brain. As aspirin is absorbed into the bloodstream it circulates through the entire body. Wherever it encounters 'prostaglandins', it will interfere with their production and thus neutralize pain. You could still be experiencing the pain, but your brain just won't get the message. This is why it is considered a cure-all for aches and pains. However, like all 'neutralizing' drugs, they will also interfere with the 'good chemicals' that the body needs to recover.

As the body is processing aspirin out of the body, 'salicin' is changed into Salicylic acid, a slightly toxic substance that will harm the stomach, liver and kidneys if taken to excess. This is why there is a warning on every package not to exceed the recommended dosage. This whole digestive process takes about 4 to 6 hours, but even taking it consistently at these intervals will eventually take its toll on the human body.[24]

Side effects from aspirin include upset stomachs, thin blood, and it is now contraindicated for fevers in children because it was found that when aspirin is given to kids with flu, chicken pox, or other viral sicknesses it can cause a potentially deadly problem known as Reye syndrome.[25] Aspirin also changes the way your kidneys make urine, it can cause some people to have trouble breathing, and in many circles is considered dangerous at very high doses. BUT, old habits die hard, and aspirin is still distributed widely and thought of as a standard remedy for those who suffer from arthritis, as well as other diseases.

A DISEASE OF ADRENAL EXHAUSTION

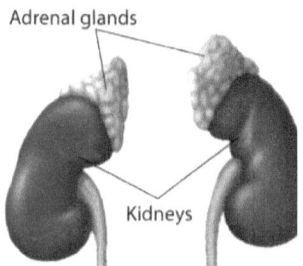

The adrenal glands produce so many chemicals that will work in conjunction with the rest of the body; getting these glands healthy is the first order of business when addressing arthritis, or any inflammatory disease. They produce all the right chemicals, in the right amount, affecting all the major organs in the body.

Getting the adrenal glands up to speed is always high on the list of things to do when entering the arena of preventative medicine as the adrenals treat several diseases, not just arthritis. This is best accomplished with specific food, vitamins and minerals, and a gradual introduction to an exercise program.

As stated before, there is no magic bullet that will cure inflammation, but by looking at a few different elements, and how they work together, we can learn a lot about what it takes to get your body on the road to recovery. Getting the adrenals back in shape takes many nutrients, with a focus on these in particular;

- Vitamin C
- Pantothenic acid; as well as all the B Vitamins
- Vitamin E
- A steady supply of protein

Improving adrenal function can take up to 2 months depending on the toxicity in the body. Because Vitamin C is used up in the detoxifying process, some people might experience detox first, before arthritic relief is found. This means that some people will experience foul smelling waste, and/ or a mild rash as their body begins to rid itself of all these toxins. This reaction is rare, but often enough that it should be mentioned. If you find this to be your case, simply lower the amount of Vitamin C you are taking to about 250 mg per day, and gradually increase it as you feel comfortable with.

By working in conjunction with their doctor, anyone can work through this to find true relief on the other side. For those that can, eating beets is a mild way to detox without the direct effects of ascorbic acid in the stomach. As always, eating detoxifying, health building foods are always better than relying completely on supplements, but then again, if we all ate right from the beginning we wouldn't be having any menacing health problems to start with. None of us are immune to that!

My critics love it when I get a cold. The only difference between my illness and everyone else's is that my illnesses only last a day or two, and don't make me to run out and purchase several expensive, toxic drugs.

Once the adrenals begin to return to normal function, they will begin to produce the necessary cortisone, as well as a host of other chemicals that will transform the arthritic body back into one that will be easy to live with. Over time, as the diet is maintained, continued improvement is seen across the board. As with many illnesses, people usually have more problems than just the primary one. Arthritis is often found in those who also suffer from bone issues; such as osteoarthritis. Adding a 2:1 mixture of Calcium and Magnesium will help to balance this out. 2-parts calcium with 1-part magnesium. This will also greatly improve sleep patterns and incontinence issues for those that have them.

VITAMIN C AND PANTOTHENIC ACID (VITAMIN B5)

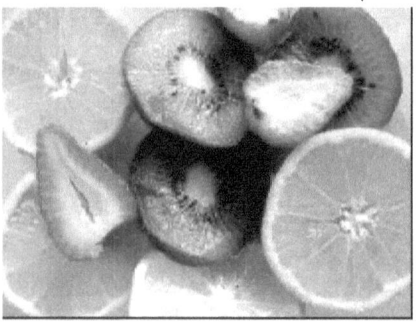

Vitamin C and Vitamin B5 are always found to be in very low amounts in the blood of people with arthritis.[26] The addition of drugs including something as simple as aspirin is also well known to increase the need for these vitamins even more.[27] One of the biggest mistakes people make is that they will take Vitamin C alone, without the Vitamin B5, or any other supporting supplements. It is important to realize that in the same way calcium needs magnesium and Vitamin D to allow it to be properly absorbed by the bones; Vitamin C needs Vitamin B5 to be properly utilized by the adrenal glands.

It is for this reason that some will also claim that taking Vitamin C can make arthritis worse; a statement that we totally disagree with and have found mountains of evidence to the contrary. Vitamin C alone will always help to halt the progression of arthritis. When added with Vitamin B5 it is known to greatly increase the positive effects of the vitamin C, and even reverse arthritis altogether.[28] Vitamin C & B5 work together much more effectively to reduce inflammation, more than if they were taken apart from one another. More study needs to be performed on the symbiotic relationship between Vitamin C and B5, but those studies that exist today will show that the combination of these two supplements has a much greater impact on those who suffer from inflammatory disease; more so than any of the other supplements available.

Since Vitamin C and Vitamin B5 are naturally occurring elements in the human diet, they will not contradict any meds being taken; and because they are water soluble, you cannot take too much. Any excess is simply excreted in the urine. Because these are water soluble, this also means that we need to eat them every day because they are not stored in the body. This easily explains why arthritis is so prevalent. Few people eat enough fresh fruit and vegetables every day; and fruit juice or fruit flavored snacks don't count.

There are still more studies showing how the side effects of cortisone and ACTH therapies are lessened when as little as 25 mg of Vitamin B5 is taken daily.[29] Like all diseases, arthritis is found more in some families, than with others, suggesting that some people might need a higher amount of Vitamin B5 than the majority of the population.[30] With so many supplemental vitamin waters available today, drinking 2-3 bottles a day is the perfect way to get your B's, and hydrate at the same time. You can't overdose on these, but you can feel a little nauseated if you eat B-vitamin tablets on an empty stomach, so be sure that you take them with at least water, if not food. It is always better to take the B Vitamins together, as a B complex supplement that includes all (8) of the B's, including;

- B1 (thiamine),
- B2 (riboflavin),
- B3 (niacin),
- B5 (pantothenic acid),
- B6,
- B7 (biotin),
- B12, and
- Folic acid

VITAMIN C

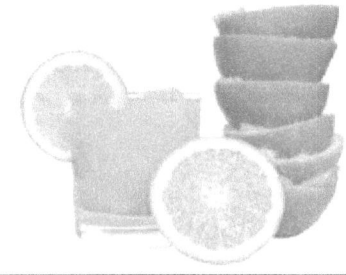

Whenever I bring up the subject of Vitamin C supplements, and all the benefits it has, I often get the standard response; "I drink orange juice." Well, this is good; but not nearly enough to combat the damage caused by disease. SO MANY diseases are influenced by Vitamin C; scurvy, cardio vascular disease, cancers, cataracts, gout, lead toxicity, increased immune system, diabetes mellitus, common cold, kidney stones, drug interactions[31], and even the simple day to day detoxification we all experience. Everyone, whether they are sick or not, should be taking some form of Vitamin C supplements every day.

HOW MUCH VITAMIN C IS ENOUGH?

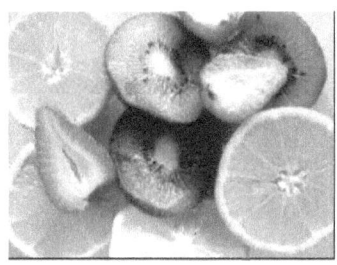

Man, guinea pigs, and some primates are the only living things that don't produce their own vitamin C, and therefore must eat it within the diet. All the other plants and animals make their own vitamin C within the liver and/ or kidneys.[32] Their metabolism will produce Vitamin C at an average rate of about 10,000 mg (10 grams) a day. When they are under stress; this will increase significantly.[33] Those living things that do not manufacture their own Vitamin C will eat approximately 13,000 mg (13 grams) per day per 150 pounds body weight.[34] This is 10 to 20 times higher than is recommended by most US nutritional guidelines.

When it comes to orange juice, the process of packaging and delivering food to the market is so involved, that by the time orange juice reaches our tables, it has lost over half of its original Vitamin C content.[35] In addition to this, 1 glass of OJ is not nearly enough to give the body what it needs on a daily basis. One cup of fresh OJ has only 124 mg (.124 grams) of vitamin C. If your OJ is not fresh, it has even less.

The information in this eBook is for those who want real relief, not a quick fix or an excuse about why vitamin C didn't work for them. If you are serious about resolving arthritis than it is going to take some real investments of time and effort to give your body what it needs. Together with your physician you will be able to stop inflammation and reverse the effects of arthritis significantly if you are willing to add supplements your diet and stay with it.

The choice between investing in vitamins and investing in synthetic drugs shouldn't be a hard one to make. Even if someone finds it hard to take 10-13 grams a day, adding 3-5 grams daily should be doable for anyone who is committed to finding relief from their arthritis pain. Even this small amount will make a big difference in your day to day activity.

There are many factors that will dictate how much each of these Vitamins is needed by each individual, but it is best to err on the side of caution, than to jump in and overload your system. There may be preexisting conditions that need to be considered so start adding your Vitamin C intake gradually, and at a pace that is tolerable for you.

It is suggested that for those who suffer from painful arthritis, taking 500mg of Vitamin C; and at least 100 mg of Vitamin B5 (Pantothenic acid) at every meal; 6 small meals a day; is a very moderate and practical way to start.

Meals don't have to be 5 courses, but just something nutritious that keeps the body's metabolism going. A banana, one apple, tomato and mozzarella cheese... as long as you are not snacking on empty calories, but using food as a vehicle to deliver nutrition, the amounts can be adjusted to suit each individual need.

The human body needs to eat fresh fruits and vegetables every day; and/or take a supplement to provide the missing nutrition. It is important to remember that there are also several nutritional elements within unprocessed food that have not been identified yet. For this reason it is always better to get your nutrition from fresh food, and supplement any additional nutrition with vitamins. By ingesting these foods naturally, we will always improve the quality of the vitamins and minerals we already know about.

Vitamin waters and a reputable multivitamin with at least the minimum recommended daily allowance (RDA) should provide a solid foundation to begin restoring health no matter how advanced arthritis is. These two elements, Vitamin C & B5, are the first line of defense for those suffering from this debilitating disease, and they should be eaten frequently throughout the day in order to bring about relief from this progressive disease.

PROTEIN AND FATTY ACIDS

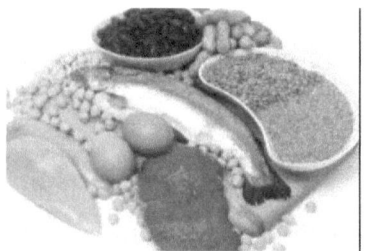

Having a decent protein intake is also important as stress can come about very quickly, causing the body to react immediately. If there is not enough protein in the diet, the body will obtain it by breaking down tissue protein if it has nothing else. Since protein is required for the body to produce ACTH[36], increasing the daily intake of it is strongly advised. Fatty acids are also needed in the utilization of protein, so these should be eaten as well. Fatty acids can be found in foods such as fish and shellfish, soy, seeds and nuts, eggs, and green leafy vegetables. It doesn't take much to give the body what it needs, so a single serving each day of any one of these things should be enough to complete the body's need for it.

Like all nutrients in the body, they have a counter part, to help assimilate, utilize, and keep in balance. Any lack of either one of these has shown a decrease in normal hormonal production.[37]

WHY SO LITTLE REFERRANCE TO VITAMINS AND MINERALS?

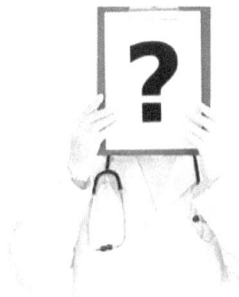

According to the MAYO clinic, Osteoarthritis is the most common form of arthritis found around the world, and there is no cure for it. It takes place when the slippery cartilage at the end of bones wears thin, and allows bone on bone contact. Since it develops with friction, it makes sense that osteoarthritis would take place in the areas that get the most use; the hands, neck, lower back, knees and hips.[38]

When looking at the MAYO Clinic's Alternative Medicine page[39], it is interesting to me how there is not even the suggestion of vitamin and minerals, but rather a very prominent, digital Flash ad for 'Celebrex'. To their credit, there is a link to the clinics alternative medicine bookstore[40] that lists (1) book, written by the MAYO Clinic's staff. It addresses herbs, botanicals, and vitamins as if they all had the same effect. As said before, herbs are fine, but it is not enough to actively build good health.

You would have to wonder? Why would such a prominent web site not make mention of vitamins, minerals, or any supplements; when there is so much evidence to the contrary? A similar format can be seen at NIH[41]; no reference to nutrition as a treatment for osteoarthritis, only yoga, acupuncture, and glucosamine. The American Arthritis Foundation will at least mention vitamins and minerals[42], but conclude their opinion with the statement that these tests are inconclusive.

There is so much documented evidence found on the internet, and in books written from the 1940's, through to the present age, documenting complete recovery from arthritis in all its forms. It is astounding to me that none of this is out for all to see. Could it be that the profits from other arthritic treatments are keeping these results under wraps deliberately? After all, it is a $128 billion industry. It has to make you wonder.

OSTEOARTHRITIS AND ITS RELATION TO MAGNESIUM, CALCIUM, AND VITAMIN E

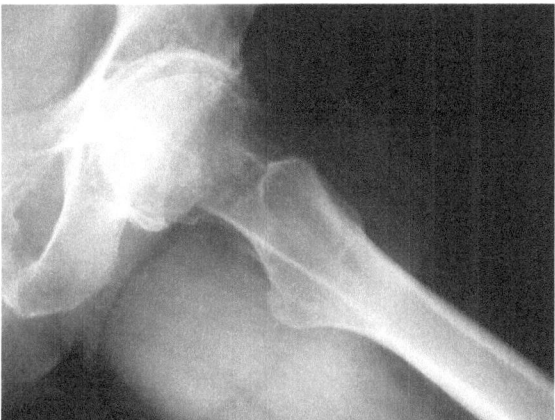

The name osteo- arthritis lets you know right away that it is a form of arthritis that involves the bone. Just like Vitamin C needs Vitamin B5 to allow it to be utilized to its full potential, calcium, vitamin D and magnesium work together in a similar way. Magnesium allows calcium to be properly deposited in the bones. Without it, magnesium deficiencies will develop, such as;

- Muscle weakness, tremors, or spasms
- Heart arrhythmia, irregular contraction, or increased heart rate
- Softening and weakening of bone
- Imbalanced blood sugar levels
- Headaches
- Elevated blood pressure

Most of the magnesium (along with calcium and phosphorous) is found inside the bone and helps to form the lattice network that provides strength. About

1/3 of it is stored in the cells and tissues waiting to be called upon when needed[43].

Magnesium also supports over 300 enzymes that are crucial to facilitating chemical reactions throughout the body. Without these enzymes, the whole network begins to come apart. Magnesium is involved with the metabolism of proteins, carbohydrates, fats, and the correct functions within genetic coding.[44] There are even some essential fuels that cannot be stored in our muscles unless there is a ready supply of magnesium to help this process take place. Magnesium is so important, that it can be found in almost every organ system in the body; including the cardiovascular system, digestive system, nervous system, muscles, kidneys, liver, the hormone-secreting glands, and the brain. Without sufficient magnesium, any one of these can falter and fail.

Like all supplements, magnesium should be taken in a balanced form, such as 2 parts calcium, with 1 part magnesium. This means that if you are taking 1000 mg of calcium, you will need about 500 mg of magnesium for the two to work together.[45]

One of the other main reasons magnesium is so important is because some people who suffer from osteoarthritis will have calcium deposits and bone spurs around their joints. When magnesium and Vitamin E are added to the diet, these are known to dissolve bone spurs within a couple of weeks.[46] Like Vitamin D, Magnesium plays a huge role in the absorption of calcium into the bones, but all the details around that will have to wait for another eBook. It is important to stay on target, and focus on how to get all arthritis, including 'osteo-'under control and heading into remission. It is important to remember that when Calcium, Magnesium, and Vitamin D are taken together, this will greatly reduce if not eliminate the development of calcium deposits around the joints. Likewise, with Vitamin E; rats with Vitamin E deficiencies will have calcium deposits in their soft tissues that increase by as much as 500%[47] when this nutrient is lacking.

Not surprisingly, all these elements are found lacking in the diets of those who suffer from this type of arthritis. These victims are also found to be under a fair amount of stress that only adds to the other deficiencies in the body.

PHOSPHEROUS

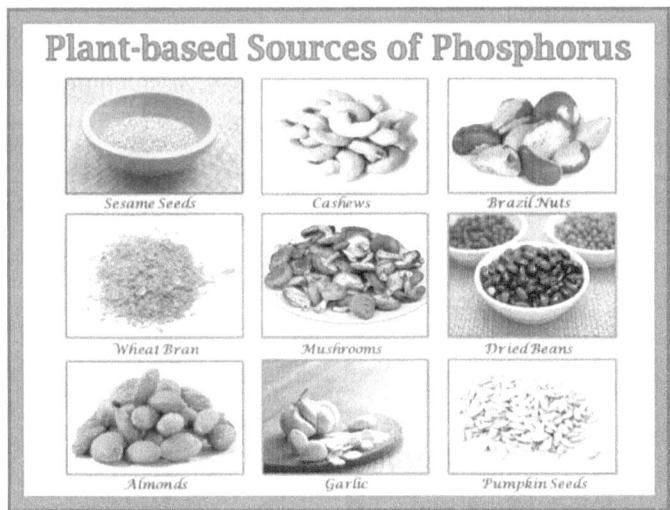

Phosphorous is an element that is often associated with bone disease, but when it comes to osteoarthritis and bone spurs, it will also come into play. It is so easy to go off on a tangent, and lose focus when talking about nutrition because so many nutritional elements work in conjunction with each other. Almost all body functions will be affected when changes are made to the diet. For this reason, I will only touch on phosphorus, and leave full comments for another one of our eBooks available on Amazon here- [48]

As stated before, when given Vitamin E and magnesium together, bone spurs are found to disappear in just a few weeks.[49] Laboratory rats kept on a diet low in calcium, but high in phosphorous developed a form of arthritis that was quickly reversed when these elements were added back into the diet. When twice as much calcium as phosphorous was given them, their fast arriving arthritis disappeared just as quickly.[50] To determine the right amounts of each, start with the right amount of calcium for you and go from there.

Arthritic patients in general, barring any outstanding existing conditions, should be taking 2 to 3 grams of calcium a day, with half as much phosphorus, and half as much magnesium, and ¼ that of Vitamin D.

Instead of trying to keep all this straight in your head, just get a reputable multi vitamin supplement, such as those from the General Nutrition Center (GNC); and add to it supplemental calcium- magnesium. These will be in the right amounts, and doses can be controlled by you. It is enough to know that it is possible to develop arthritis if you are taking in too much phosphorous, but that this can be reversed when you make sure your phosphorous intake is not more than half of your calcium intake.

SUMMARY

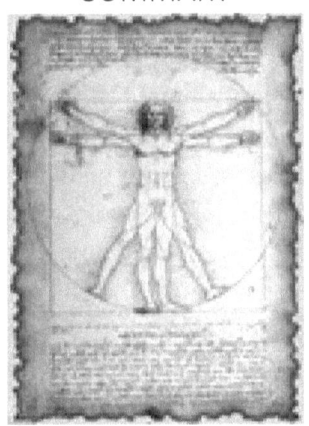

As you can see, the nutritional requirements of the body can be very complex. We hope that this eBook has made it a little easier for you. There is no 'one way' to cure arthritis. Reversing all the effects of arthritis depends on a diet rich in several nutrients, and one that includes supplements to combat stress. Like many people, the fine art of cooking is long gone from most American households, but thank God we have lots of vitamin stores, and food that can be prepared for us. If that food is real, and not processed, anyone can manage their health effectively. In summary, supplements that should be added, in order of importance are;

- 500mg Vitamin C at every meal; meals eaten in 6 small portions a day
    - A word of caution: Vitamin C is a detoxifier. If someone has had swelling for an extended amount of time, chances are their bowels are swollen, too.
    - Once the Vitamin C starts to reduce this, the body will relax, and might release some of the bacteria trapped inside the digestive tract folds.
    - This can cause a mild form of diarrhea, causing you to make more trips to the bathroom than you did before, but this is temporary. And will pass.
    - Be sure to drink lots of vitamin water to make sure you are staying hydrated and not losing these essential water-soluble nutrients.
- 100 mg of pantothenic acid at every meal, taken in the form of a B-complex that includes all the B Vitamins
- A good supply of protein; minimum 80 grams a day for men; 60 grams a day for women
- Good nutritional sources of protein include fish, meat, soy, or even 1 or 2 protein shakes a day will do the job. EAS Sports Nutrition[51] makes a great low-carb shake that is delicious, affordable (less than $1 each at Wal-Mart), and includes just about everything we need.
- Fatty Acids- these are essential oils that need to be eaten to allow for certain metabolic

functions to take place. A hand full of nuts or a tablespoon of mixed vegetable oil a day will take care of this.
- Calcium- Magnesium Supplements- 2 to 3 grams of calcium and half as much magnesium is the best balance. These can be bought in a form that is already balanced but be careful not to get calcium with Vitamin D, as vitamin D is fat soluble and will be stored in the body. Get your Vitamin D from the sun or in a multivitamin where it will be in a lessor amount. 400 units daily is an appropriate amount for most people[52].

- Vitamin E- 400 units a day[53]. Supplemental Vitamin E is essential for many metabolic processes but getting Vitamin E from food is always better. Wheat germ, green leafy vegetables, cereals, nuts, and vegetable oils are your best source; however, all Vitamin E is not created equal. Just as there are several B-Vitamins, Vitamin E also has 8 compounds of its own, making this version much better than the bottles we find in the store. Read this BLOG post to find out more -

Starting with a diet full of fresh fruits and vegetables and adding supplements to this is the best way to start reversing the effects of arthritis. If this regimen is maintained, you can expect to see your arthritis, as well as several other illnesses improve quickly until you discover that you are your old self again. Movement doesn't have to diminish with age. Just because it is common, doesn't mean it is required. There are millions of people who remain active well into their 80's and 90's, but it is not luck; these people have made the decision to give their body what it needs to perform the way it should.

Take control of your health; and you take back control over your life.

More Books Can Be Found on Amazon At;

http://www.amazon.com/author/kerriryan

Or visit our web Blog at - https://www.nutritional-therapy.us/blog to learn more about your specific condition. You can always email us directly if you have any questions-

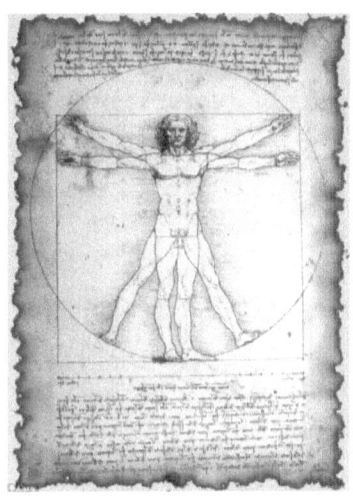

Nutritional Therapy's Medical Disclaimer;

The information on this site is not intended to be a substitute for professional medical advice, diagnosis or treatment. Each individual person has their own unique set of medical needs, and all information gathered here should be considered along with the advice of the reader's doctor. This information is intended to offer alternatives to traditional, drug related medical therapies, and the readers assume all responsibility when putting this information into effect. This information is accurate and true to the best of all authors' authority; is taken from numerous medical sources and referenced whenever possible. All content, including text, graphics, images and information, contained on or available through this publication is for general information purposes and does not take into account any other preexisting conditions. Readers will not hold NUTRITIONAL-THERAPY authors or administrators responsible for any adverse results.

NEVER DISREGARD PROFESSIONAL MEDICAL TREATMENT BECAUSE OF SOMETHING YOU HAVE READ ON OR ACCESSED THROUGH THIS MATERIAL.

Nutritional Therapy will not be responsible or liable for any course of treatment, diagnosis, or any other information, services or products that are obtained through this publication; but rather offer alternatives to those wanting to get away from prescription drugs; and those wanting to restore health naturally without them.

For more information, please contact
NutritionalTherapyUS@gmail.com

You are encouraged to report negative side effects of prescription drugs to the FDA. Visit the FDA MedWatch website;
http://www.fda.gov/Safety/MedWatch/HowToReport/default.htm or call 1-800-FDA-1088 to find out more.

[1] http://www.salans.com/en-GB/sitecore/Content/Salans/Global/Items/People/M/~/media/Assets/Salans/Publications/Pharma%20Alert_Eng.ashx, https://www.ncbi.nlm.nih.gov/pmc/articles/PMC2811591/
[2] http://www.experiment-resources.com/history-of-antibiotics.html
[3] https://www.history.com/this-day-in-history/salk-announces-polio-vaccine
[4] Let's Get Well, Davis, A., Harcourt, Brace, and World, Inc., NY 125, 1965
[5] http://www.arthritis.org/types-arthritis.php
[6] http://www.arthritis.org/facts.php
[7] http://www.arthritis.org/facts.php
[8] http://www.arthritis.org/facts.php
[9] Let's Get Well, Davis, A., Harcourt, Brace, and World, Inc., NY 125, 1965
[10] https://www.npr.org/sections/health-shots/2014/09/22/349875448/best-to-not-sweat-the-small-stuff-because-it-could-kill-you
[11] http://www.arthritis.org/principles-arthritis-management.php
[12] https://en.wikipedia.org/wiki/Biopsychosocial_model
[13] http://www.arthritis.org/understanding-arthritis.php
[14] http://www.ncbi.nlm.nih.gov/pmc/articles/PMC372541/
[15] http://www.hss.edu/conditions_steroid-side-effects-how-to-reduce-corticosteroid-side-effects.asp
[16] https://www.mayoclinic.org/tests-procedures/cortisone-shots/about/pac-20384794
[17] http://en.wikipedia.org/wiki/Adrenocorticotropic_hormone
[18] http://www.ncbi.nlm.nih.gov/pmc/articles/PMC1627020/
[19] http://www.arthritis.org/understanding-arthritis.php
[20] http://www.experiment-resources.com/history-of-antibiotics.html
[21] http://www.experiment-resources.com/history-of-antibiotics.html

[22] http://www.arthritis.org/principles-arthritis-management.php
[23] http://www.ncbi.nlm.nih.gov/pmc/articles/PMC1627020/
[24] http://health.howstuffworks.com/medicine/medication/aspirin1.htm
[25] http://health.howstuffworks.com/medicine/medication/aspirin4.htm
[26] Morgan, A.F., J. Bio. Chem. 195, 583, 1952,
[27] Eising,L.J., Bone Joint Surgery, 452, 69, 1963, Linus Pauling Institute; http://lpi.oregonstate.edu/infocenter/vitamins/vitaminC - 'drug interactions'
[28] Barboriak, J.J., et al, J Nutrition 63, 601, 1957
[29] Oppenheimer, E.H., et al., Bull. John's Hopkins Hosp., 107, 297, 1960; Lamont-Havers, R.W., Borden's Rev. Nutritional Response, 24, 1, 15, 1963; Zucker,T.A., Am. J. Clin. Nutrition, 6, 65, 1958;
[30] Wlliams, R.J., Biomedical Individuality, Wiley, N.Y.
[31] http://lpi.oregonstate.edu/infocenter/vitamins/vitaminC/
[32] http://en.wikipedia.org/wiki/Vitamin_C 'Biosynthesis in Diff. Species'
[33] http://www.seanet.com/~alexs/ascorbate/197x/stone-i-orthomol_psych-1979-v8-n2-p58.htm
[34] http://www.seanet.com/~alexs/ascorbate/197x/stone-i-orthomol_psych-1979-v8-n2-p58.htm
[35] http://www.ultimatecitrus.com/vitaminc.html
[36] Tui, C.J., Clinical Nutrition, 1, 232
[37] Glatzel, H., Nutrition Abstract (Rev.1964), 34, 507
[38] http://www.mayoclinic.com/health/osteoarthritis/DS00019
[39] http://www.mayoclinic.com/health/osteoarthritis/DS00019/DSECTION=alternative-medicine
[40] https://store.mayoclinic.com/products/books/Details.cfm?mpid=61&trkid=21242S198705060

[41] http://www.ncbi.nlm.nih.gov/pubmedhealth/PMH0001460/
[42] http://www.arthritis.org/disease-center.php?disease_id=32&df=treatments
[43] http://www.ncbi.nlm.nih.gov/pubmed/3970732
[44] http://www.whfoods.com/genpage.php?tname=nutrient&dbid=75
[45] http://www.livestrong.com/article/517661-relationship-between-calcium-magnesium/
[46] MacIntyre, I., et al., BioChem. J., 70,465,1958; Maynard, L.A., et al., J. Nutrition, 64, 85,1958; Bruce, G.E., et al., J. of Nutrition, 76,23, 1962; Steiner, A.J., Applied Nutrition, 16, 125, 1963
[47] Morgales, S., et al., J. Biol. Chem., 124, 767, 1938; Ames, S.R., J. Biol. Chem., 169, 503, 1947
[48] http://www.amazon.com/Kerri-Ryan/e/B006P0FZUE/ref=ntt_athr_dp_pel_1
[49] Ames, S.R., J. Biol. Chem., 169, 503, 1947; Morgales, S., et al., J. Biol. Chem., 124, 767, 1938
[50] Hogan, A.G., et al., J. Nutrition, 41, 203, 1950
[51] http://eas.com/product/advantedge-carb-control-ready-to-drink
[52] http://www.doctoroz.com/videos/daily-dose-vitamin-d
[53] http://www.sciencedaily.com/releases/2008/10/081030144718.htm